## Wrinkle Prevention

# Beautiful Skin in 7 Days

Lerone E. Abrams

ISBN: 0988890402
ISBN-13: 978-0-9888904-0-4

WRINKLE PREVENTION: *Beautiful Skin In 7 Days*



| | |
|---|---|
| Author: | Lerone E. Abrams |
| Editor: | Winslow Eliot |
| Cover Design & Art: | Jennifer Fitzgerald |
| Published by: | Lerone E. Abrams |

Composed and printed in the United States of America

Version: 2012.7

# CONTENTS

# Preface

I wrote this book because I saw the benefits of healthy living, which includes diets, nutritional supplements, topical applications and stress management. At a young age of 24 I had worked several jobs simultaneously, racking up 18 and 20 hour days. I was eating fast food every day, and was stressed out of my mind, which wreaked havoc on my appearance. I ended up with bags under my eyes, skin discolorations from pimples, and premature wrinkles. By accident, I got sick and decided to take some supplements. To my surprise, my health and energy improved drastically as well as my skin. But what really hooked me on this new way of life was the compliments I received from family and friends. "You look good Lee. You're a handsome young man, you take care of yourself well." After receiving these compliments and gaining newfound attention, I was motivated to discover as much as I could about natural health. I subsequently devoted myself to the health industry, working for one of the top nutritional stores in America, and researching skin care, nutrition, and diet.

In this book you will find techniques and strategies that greatly improve your appearance. Using the techniques provided will be to your great advantage. Now is the time to start taking care of your skin: no more excuses. If you already have wrinkles-that's fine, we will diminish them or get rid of them altogether.

I would like to thank my parents Hazel and Clarence Abrams for their unconditional love and support through the writing of this book. I would also like to thank Holly Kuntz for her help and unwavering support. And the list is too long to write, but to all my family and friends who have encouraged me and eagerly awaited this book, thank you!

*Wrinkle Prevention: Beautiful Skin in 7 days* took 2 ½ years to write. The challenge was to provide a clear and simple guide, yet one flexible enough to cover a variety of issues related to anti-wrinkle therapy and gaining beautiful skin.

The techniques and suggestions contained within these pages are for women ages 18 to 40, but anyone can benefit from the suggestions and insights offered.

# Introduction

Thank you for allowing me the opportunity to provide valuable insights and solutions to meet your skin care needs. In this book you will find information, techniques, products, and insights that will forever change your skin for the better.

I was watching *The Today Show* one morning and on this particular episode, the female anchors went without makeup for the day. Though they are attractive women, it was shocking how weathered their skin looked, but what was most shocking was the belief that caked-on makeup was necessary for them to look their best. The truth is your skin should be beautiful with or without makeup, and I will show you how.

To prevent wrinkles and bad skin, proper nutrition and diet are necessary: many women don't realize this. They smoke, drink alcohol, eat fast food, exercise infrequently, don't use moisturizers, and wear excessive makeup to cover it all up. The result is that their skin ages prematurely. However, you don't have to have weathered and dull skin. Using the techniques offered here will eliminate the need to wear any makeup at all. Your skin will glow - from the inside out. This book is written for anyone who wants to look his or her best. I will show you scientific and proven methods to eliminate and reduce wrinkles. If you follow the regimen prescribed here, you'll find that your skin will glow; it will appear strong, radiant, vibrant, and lively.

Before you start any skin care regimens or treatment, or undergo any invasive therapy, follow the techniques in this book. It will save you endless amount of time, energy, and money.

## *Philosophy*

The philosophy of this book is simple: Natural First. That means I will recommend to you the most natural and healthy ways to improve your skin, before recommending any invasive treatments. That is my first bias as it relates skincare. My second bias is that these methods, natural or procedural, must work. If a new technology of method shows promise I will inform you. Natural products are less likely to cause harm to your skin or have adverse side effects.

Many women, as soon as they start to notice the signs of aging, go and visit their dermatologist, which is commendable. The dermatologist then prescribes a few drugs, sometimes steroids for acne and scars, dermal fillers for wrinkles, and a face lift for sagging skin. The dermatologists do not ask about your diet, your supplements intake, or your workout routine: these crucial questions never come up. In itself, the process your dermatologist uses isn't wrong *per se*, because that is how they were trained. However, the basic assumptions and methods are flawed. There is a better way: the holistic treatment of the entire human being, not just prescribing medication and surgeries. The training these doctors receive relies heavily on the prescription of drugs and invasive procedures that cause harm to your body. Doctors have a bias of prescribing drugs and invasive treatments before natural remedies are explored, whereas my bias is natural treatments first.

I am in no way bashing these doctors, also known as dermatologists, who treat skin issues, and plastic surgeons, the ones who perform invasive treatments, because they are highly trained individuals with expertise in their fields. The history of plastic surgery in America goes back to 1920s, after World War I, many soldiers came back home with horrific injuries, such as blown off noses, eye loss, and other terrible facial and bodily disfigurements. For these injuries, gifted, smart, and intelligent surgeons are needed to carry out these difficult corrective surgeries, and I applaud them for doing so.

However, when I hear of women getting Botox injections, skin peels, face lifts, and other invasive treatments to fix such things as fine lines, wrinkles, age spots, and dullness, I say to myself: "Hold on, wait a minute! Shouldn't natural remedies be explored first? Do these people know that there are natural remedies that work? Do they know that these invasive therapies could have long-lasting, nasty side effects?

My motivation behind writing this book is to show you the natural techniques that work for your skin.

## *How to use this book*

First, take the questionnaire, which identifies your skin type. Afterward, go to the corresponding chapter that contains the information on your skin type and read the recommendations. Get a pen or pencil and a journal or notepad to write down what you've learned. Then read the rest of the chapters and follow the guidelines. It's also helpful to read the chapters containing other skin types, because you might have more than one skin type, because skin types change with time.

After you have achieved results, send me an email so I can follow up with suggestions and answer questions you may have.

Thank you, and enjoy your beautiful skin to come!

# Your Skin

Certain cultures say the face reflects the soul, and if that is true, in order to best complement your face, great skin is required. But, if your face reflects your soul, then your skin reflects your emotions: how you eat, sleep, exercise, think, and your overall habits. Your habits ultimately affect the health of your skin, internally and externally.

The skin is the largest organ in the body, and at times can be the most neglected. Skin filters waste from the body and protects other organs from damage. There are three layers to the skin: epidermis, dermis, and hypodermis.

The epidermis is the outermost layer of the skin. It is the first protector of the body; it prevents many of the sun's harmful rays from reaching other organs and tissue. These rays are called the ultraviolet radioactive long range rays (UVA) and the ultraviolet radioactive short range rays (UVB). The UVA rays travel through the epidermis and reach all the way to the hypodermis. UVA rays penetration can cause melanoma, the most dangerous form of skin cancer. The epidermis stops the UVB rays from the sun, but you pay the price by getting burned on its surface. As a result, UVB rays are usually responsible for basal cell and squamous cell cancers.

The dermis is the middle layer of the skin. The dermis is made up of connective tissue. It contains the sebaceous glands, which are responsible for providing the skin's natural oil, called sebum. It also contains the sweat glands and blood vessels. These sweat glands work to cool the body and excrete toxins, while the blood vessels work to circulate nutrients and oxygen the skin needs.

The hypodermis is the innermost layer of the skin. It attaches the upper layers of the skin to the rest of your body. It is composed of connective tissue, elastin, and fatty tissue. Around 50 percent of this skin is made up of fatty tissue that decreases with age.

**Pick an area or areas of the face you want to see improved and write it down. If you need help, use the list of common skin problems on the next page. Write down the problematic areas and then label them with today's date.**

Pick and write down the area you would like to see improved.

- ☐ Oily skin
- ☐ Dry patches
- ☐ Scars
- ☐ Lines at the corner of mouth
- ☐ Bags under eyes
- ☐ Discolorations
- ☐ Tone
- ☐ Smoothness
- ☐ Acne
- ☐ Blotchiness

If possible, take your picture and also date it with today's date.

# Skin Types

Some doctors and skin experts say there are no skin types. Some say there are two to three main skin types, while others have gone all the way up to 16 skin types. These skin types typically include oily, dry, sensitive, hyper pigmentation, dark, and pale skin. The truth is there are several different skin types, and the number and definition varies depending on whether you're speaking with a doctor, a cosmetician, esthetician, or a marketer for a cosmetic company.

First, let's define what a skin type is. *A skin type is any skin that is categorized by melanin content, oil production, and/or by a prevalent or consistent condition of the skin: color, texture, and other conditions.* Besides melanin content which is usually stable, other aspects of your skin type usually change throughout your life, because of age and many other factors.

The fact is that the traditional skin types - oily, dry, and combination - are directly affected by our diet, hormones, stress, contraceptives, weather, and all sorts of other daily occurrences. This means that one day your skin can be oily and the next it can be dry. Puberty and menstruation can cause the skin to be more oily than usual, since hormones play a big role in the traditional skin type characterizations. A solution? Zinc and Vitamin A help to balance hormones, which in turn regulates oil distribution to the skin, and stops acne. Literally, those two supplements can cause oily skin to turn normal.

As we've said, there are several different skin types. We have organized skin types as followed the main skin types are oily, dry, normal, and combination. The secondary skin types or skin conditions are sensitive, pigmented, acne, rosacea, eczema, and your skin's melanin content (skin color). It is possible to have a combination of the main skin types with one or more of the secondary skin types. For example oily- and acne-prone skin types usually occur together because many times the oil is trapped under the skin and mixed with hair and bacteria, which causes a blackheads and pimples. Dry skin accompanied with acne also occurs, although less commonly.

### Determining Your Skin Type

Get a pen or pencil and in your journal, write My Skin Type and underline it.

Then write the number one.

First we are going to determine your general skin type:

### Section I. General Skin Type: Oily, Dry, Normal, or Combination

Wash your face and wait an hour.

A) Oily

B) Dry

C) Oily in certain spots and dry in others

D) Appropriately balanced, with no overly oily or ashy areas

For further confirmation: take a tissue and wipe your skin.

A) If oil rubs off on tissue, your skin is oily

B) If skin cells rub off on tissue, your skin is dry

C) If nothing rubs off, your skin is normal

D) If oil comes off the T-Zone or other parts, then you have combination skin

Write down your answer.

**Section II. Predisposed wrinkled or thinned skin, Pigmented, or Acne**

1) Do you have pale skin, blond hair, and blue eyes?

Yes or No

2) Do your parents have wrinkles, and if so, when did they start to get them (20s, 30s, or 40s)?

Yes or No

3) Is your skin dry and does it crack easily?

Yes or No

4) a. Do you currently have wrinkles?

b. If so, are you in your 20s, or early 30s?

If you answered yes to two or more questions, then you have predisposed thin skin or wrinkled skin type.

If you answered yes just to question four, you most likely have premature wrinkling due to sun damage, stress, or poor skin care.

## Section III - Pigmentation

5) Does your skin have scars, spots, freckles, or marks from razor bumps?

6) On your face, are there different shades of colors in different spots?

7) Are you under the age of thirty with age spots?

If you answer yes to any of these questions, you have pigmented skin.

## Section IV - Sensitivity in Your Skin

8) Does your skin react to moisturizers or facial care products?

9) Is your skin generally red, pimple-prone, or prone to rashes or outbreaks of dermatitis?

10) Does your skin break out from jewelry and sun exposure?

11) Do your parents suffer from any skin disorder, such as rosacea, psoriasis, eczema,

redness, or skin inflammation?

If you answered yes to two of these questions, you have sensitive skin type.

If you answered yes to question 10 or 11, it is highly probable your skin is sensitive.

***Now go to the relevant section that pertains to your needs. Skin types usually occur in combination, so you may have a combination of several skin types.***

## *I. Normal skin*

Normal skin has an adequate balance of oil and water. You should definitely wear a moisturizer and sunblock to maintain healthy skin and block sun rays from aging your skin. This is the kind of skin you are born with until puberty. It is soft, smooth, and wrinkle-free. If your skin currently fits this description, you can be very glad and happy. Some may say you need stronger products to penetrate your skin, or products that contain alcohol to carry ingredients deep into to the skin. Absolutely do not do it! Your skin has something called NMF, or Natural Moisturizing Factor, which is a natural film that covers your face. Because of this, at times your face might look slightly oily. Work with your natural oils, not against them.

*Recommendation:*

Your goal should be to maintain this skin type. Drink 8 glasses of water a day. Wear sunscreen of at least 15 SPF and use a lotion or moisturizer underneath to keep a barrier between your sunblock and your skin.

## *II. Combination skin*

Regardless of the bad press it receives for being oily and dry at the same time, it is not as bad as it seems. The skin is usually slightly oily in the T-zone and slightly dry on the cheeks. At times your skin could be dry on one day and oily on the next. Climate changes and the weather have a lot to do with this.

*Recommendation:*

Wash oily areas with warm water and normal or dry areas in cool to cold water. This is a targeted approach that will lock-in moisture and oils in the dry areas of the skin, while reducing excessive oils in oily areas. For oily sections of the skin use Carlson Face wash soap, and on normal and dry areas use Jason's ester C soap.

Reminder: The T-zone is usually oily on the forehead and the cheeks are either normal or dry.

Use the astringent witch hazel for both oily and dry areas. If your skin is still oily after using witch hazel for a week, try tea tree-oil instead which is a stronger solution. Apply talcum powder on the nose or on areas of the face that produce the most oil. It is not uncommon for your skin to be dry one day and oily the next. Weather, environment, menstrual cycle, diet and nutrition all have an effect on your skin. Also, vitamin A facial gel can be used on your entire face because it is grease-free but provides moisture.

### *III. Dry skin*

Dry skin wrinkles more easily than oily skin. The reason is that dry skin loses oil, which in turn causes water within skin cells to dissipate. Once the moisture of the skin is gone, the skin is more susceptible to cracking, and once facial expressions are made, the skin doesn't have the suppleness to push out the lines caused by those facial expressions. Having dry skin makes you much more susceptible to developing thin and wrinkled skin. If you're Caucasian or your skin is dry, regardless of your age, you have to start caring for your dry skin immediately.

*Recommendation:*

Drink 8 glasses of water every day, take essential fatty acids, primrose oil, or fish oil. Use oil based soaps and other gentle cleansers. Apply to face and then rinse with warm water. Use flora water as a toner; spray it on, then apply moisturizer shortly before it dries. Use a moisturizer that contains aloe vera, elastin, or collagen.

At night, use a heavier oil-based moisturizer. These moisturizers should contain haluranoic acid, collagen cream, elastin cream, vegetable glycerin, vitamin E, and panthenol. Avoid petroleum and mineral oil. Wash face in cool to cold water.

### *IV. Oily skin*

This may possibly be the best skin type to have, more so as you get older (35 and up), even better than normal skin. As you get older, your skin tends to dry and become thinner. Black and Mediterranean women produce more oil on their skin and this causes them to resist wrinkles well into their 50s and 60s. Oily skin is caused by over-production of sebum, the skin's natural oil. Oily skin is less susceptible to wrinkling than dry skin because the extra oils lubricate the skin and keep in more moisture. However, just because your skin is oily doesn't mean your skin has adequate amounts of moisture. Moisture is the water within your skin cell. The oil of your skin locks in the water within the skin cells. Sebum works in tandem with water to keep your skin healthy. Use an oil-free moisturizer, even if you have oily skin, because it supplies your skin with moisture and water that the skin needs, and it will protect against free radical damage if the moisturizer contains vitamin A, C, or E, or a combination of all three. It will even protect against the chemicals in sunscreens. There is a correlation between oily skin and acne breakouts. However, the lubrication helps with protecting the skin from UVA rays, cracking, and formation of wrinkles. Work with your skin; you have an advantage in the prevention of wrinkling as you get older, so use it. If your skin is a little oily, use a tissue and wipe off the oil, then apply powder. In many ways, the oily skin type is the preferred type as you get older.

*Recommendations*:

Keep skin clean, use products with mild tea tree oil or benzoyl peroxide of .05%, and use a clay or mud mask to take away excessive oils 2 to 3 times a week. Use zinc to regulate oil secretion. Use lemon and water once or twice a day. Use talcum powder to blot oil secretion and use an astringent such as witch hazel to absorb oil. Wash face in warm to very warm water.

### *V. Sensitive Skin*

The positives of this skin type are that skin care products will work at a faster pace than on any other skin type; however, you're going to have to be more vigilant about what you eat, wear, and put on your skin. If your sheets have bacteria, that can affect your skin; if you wear the same shirt twice in a row, that can cause a breakout. Other contributors to sensitive skin: cologne, perfume, a backed-up colon, stress, nutritional imbalance, low immune function, and an underlying sickness. Sensitive skin is prone to break-outs, inflammation, and infection caused by fragrances and preservatives in skin care products, especially products that contain a variety of ingredients.

*Recommendations*:

Use gentle oils, preferably your products should contain very little to no fragrances and preservatives. Keep your skin clean, and wear clothes once and then wash, because dead skin cells, sweat, and bacteria on clothes will irritate your skin. Keep a record of the foods you eat, because they may irritate your skin. Common food allergens are peanuts, peanut butter, bee products, soy products, and oranges.

### *VI. Pigmented*

Highly pigmented skin heals with scars, spots, and freckles. You should be aware of products that may cause irritation or bumps. This skin type is usually prevalent in African Americans, Asians,

Hispanics, and people of Mediterranean descent. People of these races have more melanin in their skin than Caucasians and Nordic Europeans. The positives with this skin type are that the melanin blocks the sun's rays and provides protection for the skin. This means less wrinkling and sun damage. The bad news is that you are more likely to suffer from skin inflammation and scarring. The reason for this is that the extra melanin forms excessive kelatus (a substance used to heal the skin), causing a thick scar. African Americans, who have the greatest amount of melanin, should never do skin peels or cosmetic procedures that require cutting of the skin. Asians, Hispanics, and Mediterranean people don't have as much melanin as African Americans, but they also should be wary of invasive treatments. Keep vitamin E and/or soy lotions on hand for such occurrences.

*Recommendations*:

Avoid picking at pimples and invasive cosmetic procedures. Use vitamin E on marks, from the neck down. If you are a sensitive skin type, use cocoa butter with vitamin E. Over-the-counter hydrocortisone creams are also good for marks. Use for a week, stop, and then continue use. Use sunscreen to prevent the formation of age spots and freckles from occurring. Products containing soy, niacin, and tyrosinase are good for reducing and preventing discolorations of the skin.

### *VII. Predisposed thin/wrinkled skin*

This skin type is mostly found in fairer skin types. Usually, the older you get, the thinner the dermis gets, and the stratum corme, which is the outermost layer of the epidermis, increases in thickness due to dead skin cells. After age 25, your skin does not replenish itself at the same rate it did when you were younger. Your skin begins to lose moisture and oil. If you are Caucasian or have very pale skin, blond hair, and blue eyes, you are predisposed to having thinner skin. Look at pictures of your mother, father, and their parents; if possible, ask your parents when they started to notice wrinkles.

*Recommendations:*

Use chondroitin and MSM sulfate to help get rid of premature wrinkles in your 20s and 30s. Stay out of the sun, because it reduces moisture in the skin and creates free radical damage. Always keep your face moisturized. Eat antioxidant rich foods and take the vitamin supplements recommended in the supplement section of this book.

## VIII. Acne

Acne may occur in combination with other skin types. It is most prevalent in sensitive and oily skin. The acne skin type is characterized by constant breakouts of acne, blackheads, whiteheads, and clogged pores. The sebaceous gland produces a natural oil called sebum. When trapped by blocked pores, sebum mixes with hair follicles, dirt, and bacteria, and causes breakouts. This occurs most commonly during puberty. Many women also experience premenstrual breakouts.

*Recommendations:*

Keep skin clean and wear clothes once. In the event of a breakout, rub tea tree oil, diluted with water, on the affected area.

Oftentimes skin types are spoken of in a manner of being stable and unchangeable. However, that perception is false. Your skin type *can* change. It is affected by your diet, climate, exposure to sun, stress, excessive washing, and change in hormones. Zinc and vitamin A supplements can change a person's skin type from oily to normal. Essential fatty acids can cause dry skin to become lubricated.

Pigmentation is usually stable with age; however, a person with pigmented skin is more likely to develop age spots from repeated unprotected exposure to the sun's rays. There are certain supplements that can increase the melanin in your skin, such as carotene and tyrosine - even the sun.

# Process of Aging

Aging is the process of growing and then ultimately passing over. For years, scientists have been trying to figure out why we age and what we can do to slow down the process. We can't live forever, but believe me the fountain of youth is here. As we become more advanced, so too will our ability to live longer, healthier lives. We have discovered several aspects of the fountain of youth that will slow down the aging process and improve our quality of life. Here are some suggestions and insights, which, if followed, will improve your health and give you a more youthful appearance.

The fountain of youth is your mind, healthy eating, exercise, supplementation, doctor visits, and maintenance.

There are several theories that attempt to explain why we age. We are going to cover eight of them.

***Active Aging*:**

A protein has been found in people who have aged prematurely, called progeria, Progeria is the disease in which people age extensively beyond their chronological age. It was found that the protein progerin was the culprit. Now in recent studies scientists have found that the protein progerin is also activated as we get older in people without the disease. It might explain why someone may seem to age over night or age beyond his or her years. Progeria are also found in people without the disease, though in smaller amounts. As telomere decreases progerin increases with age.

### *DNA/Genetic Theory:*

This theory states that our genes are responsible for the rate at which we age. Genes are responsible for hair and eye color, height, and every other part of the physical being. There is a high correlation between genes and longevity. But external forces such as stress, poor diet, environmental pollutants, and the sun's rays can damage our DNA and genes. This stops or slows down the body's ability to repair or rejuvenate itself.

### *Cell metabolic theory:*

Eat less, live long, eat five small meals a day. There are two hypotheses behind this theory. The first is that if less calories are consumed, cell division will slow down. This was found in animal studies. The second hypothesis states that if fewer calories are consumed, then less free radical damage will occur from the oxidation. Oxidation is the result of the creation of energy from digested food.

### *Cross Linking/Glucose/Sugar Theory:*

This theory states that sugars such as glucose bind or cross links with proteins. These proteins then cross links with other proteins, which damages surrounding tissue and causes aging. The process also causes free radicals to form and it stops certain processes that are important for the life of a healthy cell.

### *Hormone Theory/Hormonal Aging:*

The hypothymus, or the pituitary gland, stops regulating hormones and produces less and less hormones, and this causes aging. Some of these hormones are HGH and testosterone. HGH and testosterone repair tissue, builds muscle, as well as bones. After production of these hormones decreases, our bodies can no longer build muscle or bone effectively. Testosterone also is responsible for keeping skin strong and the overall vitality of the body. (I recommend hormone-replacement therapy for people in their 40s and up. If you use hormone-replacement therapy while the body still produces these hormones, there is a strong likelihood that your body will decrease or stop producing these hormones altogether. Go to your physician's office and get tested for hormone deficiencies.)

### *Free Radical/Oxidation Theory:*

As we get older, free radicals increase, while at the same time we produce decreasing amounts of antioxidants to fight off a growing number of free radicals. These free radicals harm and destroy cells, proteins, DNA, and RNA, and this results in aging. Free radical damage can also lead to cancer.

### *Immune Theory:*

As we get older, the immune systems decreases in effectiveness and begins attacking itself. The immune system is responsible for fighting off the common cold, flu, infection, and diseases. When the body gets older, the immune system cannot fight off these things effectively, while protective immune cells continue to decrease with age.

***Stem Cell Theory:***

As we age, we produce fewer stem cells. Stem cells repair and grow tissue. If we were to replace the lost stem cells, we would live longer. The body then acquires cells that are malfunctioning in tissue such as in the skin, causing aging. Stem cells have the ability to turn into other body cells. This may be the most controversial theory of them all, not because the theory isn't sound, but because certain religious and political groups are strongly against the use of stem cells since they can be harvested from human embryos.

We have combined all these theories to give you the best proven methods for staying healthy, youthful, and vibrant. Most likely, one or all of these theories contribute to the aging process. It is my view that all these theories provide viable explanations for the aging process. The proven methods I discuss in this book will help you protect yourself from many of the factors that cause aging.

# Wrinkles

As we age, our skin begins to lose its suppleness and elasticity. As a result, it becomes dryer and thinner. Smile lines and marks from other facial expressions remain on the face. When the skin still had its suppleness and elasticity, these lines would disappear immediately. As we age, these lines deepen and become more noticeable.

The aging process is active. Scientists recently found that progeria, the protein that causes premature aging, is also active in the normal aging process. As we get older, our skin begins to produce larger amounts of free radicals, which are usually destroyed by antioxidants within the skin cells. However, at this stage, the number of antioxidants in the skin is decreasing, while the number of free radicals is increasing. The free radicals then roam the skin, damaging collagen, connective tissue, proteins, and other skin cells. This damage causes the skin to become inflamed, which further deteriorates the fabric of the skin. It is a combination of these processes that causes wrinkles. In addition, as we age, our skin becomes dryer, which worsens the appearance of wrinkles.

The first signs of wrinkles usually appear around the eyes and mouth. The lines around the mouth have a more pronounced effect on your appearance than anywhere else on your face. The next affected areas are the cheeks and lips. As we go through our daily routine, our skin is affected by the sun, environmental pollutants, lack of nutrition, bad diet, and smoking. Harm from these pollutants can be reversed, but it is going to take patience to hold on to results and continue to develop beautiful, radiant skin.

Sun exposure is thought by many to be the main culprit when it comes to skin damage and wrinkles. The sun dries the skin out and its UVA rays cause free radical damage on a cellular level. Fair-skinned people are especially affected by the sun's rays. If you plan to be out in the sun, it's crucial that you wear sunblock. At all costs, protect your skin from the sun, even if it means you won't get your daily dose of vitamin D3, which you can always obtain in supplement form. Most of what we think is caused by aging is actually caused by the sun and its harmful UVA rays. Even when the day is dark, rainy, or cloudy, these UVA rays are still present in the atmosphere and can have the same effect on your skin. The UVA rays destroy the tissue that keeps the skin firm, plump, and flexible. When the skin tissue is bathed by these rays, over time, the elasticity is broken down, causing wrinkles. Protect yourself with sunblock; use a broad range of sunblocks that contain zinc oxide and titanium dioxide.

- Additional causes of wrinkles: genes, stress, diet, habit, environment, and improper skin cosmetics.

- In the following chapters I will give you in-depth instructions on how to get rid of and protect against wrinkles.

# Stress

Stress is a psychological, emotional, and physiological response to events and things that have happened to us that is perceived in a negative way. It affects almost all of us at some time and continues as long as we live. Stress wreaks havoc on your health and skin. It causes cortisol to be released into the system, which prompts the immune system to over-function. Some symptoms of stress may include ulcers, frequent illness, sleeplessness, excessive sleep, or low energy. These are all signs that your immune system is down. When your immune system is down, it makes you more susceptible to the effects of bags under the eyes, crow's feet, blanched skin, breakouts, and UVA rays. In order to protect the skin, find ways to reduce stress.

Some supplements that are good for relieving stress are: vitamin B, vitamin C, melatonin, SAM-e, and St. John's wort. Another technique for reducing stress is relaxing. Practice deep breathing exercises, hold your breath, clench your muscles tight, and then let go and breathe. Do this several times a day this will teach you how to control high tension and relax.

# Cleanses

The first step to great skin is to cleanse your body of waste and toxins. There are several ways to do this, fasting is a good way to give your body's digestive tract a rest and to cleanse your colon. A simple fasting technique is to drink lemon water for three days along with two quarts of water per day. For the lemon water, use one half to a whole lemon, peeled and blended with 16 ounces of water. Limit meals to one a day. Do a trial run when you have a day off. Fasting can take some getting used to, and if your body isn't accustomed to it, you may become tired and have hunger pains initially. It is highly recommended that you start when you are in a comfortable environment. An alternative plan for cleaning is to invest in psyllium husk pills or powder and add it to a cup of juice to help with your daily motion.

*Colon*

This is the most basic of cleanses. Technically, every bowel movement can be considered a colon cleanse. Most likely, it is not thorough enough. It is estimated that 80 percent of diseases start in the colon. This can be easily overlooked because of our busy lives, and only brought to light when we need to lose weight, are constipated, or a cleanse that is recommended by a physician. A colon cleanse is essential for good skin care. When your colon is in its optimal state, your skin will be vibrant and healthy.

Suggested products: use psyllium husk or lemon water. Men: use one lemon with 16 ounces of water. Women: use half a lemon with 16 ounces of water.

*Blood, Kidney, & Liver*

The kidney and the liver are responsible for filtering toxins out of the blood. The foods we eat today contain many toxins, parasites, hormones, and steroids. These negatively affect our organs, bodies, and skin. Steroids may cause our bodies to produce excess oil, retain toxins in the skin, and encourage harmful organisms to grow in the body. Steroids, pesticides, and even prescribed medications can be taxing on the liver and kidney. A cleanse of the liver and kidney will help them to function more effectively, reducing the skin's need to filter the body's waste.

Suggested products: Red clover, celery & parsley, cranberries, dandelion root, hydrangea, and uva ursi.

*Urinary Tract Cleanse*

This cleanse works by urinating out the impurities in your body that cause skin breakouts and irritation. Excessive yeast or candidiasis cause inflammation, which is not just bad for your body, but bad for your skin. A urinary tract cleanse is good for cleansing the body of candidiasis.

Suggested products: Black cherry, celery & parsley, cranberries, hydrangea, and uva ursi.

*Fasting*

This is best way to cleanse the body if you have time and capability. Fasting has been around since biblical times, and has been incorporated into every major religion today. Fasting cleanses your system while giving your digestive tract a rest. One way to fast is by juicing, which is a good way to obtain nutrients. Juicing involves the blending of fruits and/or vegetables and then the extraction of the fiber. Blending is also a good way to get nutrients, however the fiber is still intact from the fruits or vegetables. For cleansing purposes blending is best because the fiber facilitates digestion. Whereas, juicing is better for obtaining nutrients.

# Diet

The second step to achieving beautiful skin is nutrition. Nutrition is arguably the most important step in maintaining young, healthy skin. It works from the inside out. Eat lots of raw or lightly steamed vegetables to retain nutritional content. The vegetables you eat should have a range of different colors, such as red, green, and orange. Some of these vegetables include broccoli, cabbage, tomatoes, cauliflower, green beans, and carrots. A plate full of colors is nature's way of saying you are on the right track. The different colors in these vegetables represent phytochemicals and vitamins, which are powerful agents for the body. These phytochemicals and vitamins enable the body to slow down the aging process and stave off disease.

Eat a balanced diet that includes a variety of fruits and vegetables, preferably raw, to provide your skin with the nutrients it needs. Also, eat whole grains, seeds, nuts, and legumes.

Drink at least 2 quarts of water every day, even if you don't feel thirsty. This will help to keep the skin hydrated, flush away toxins, and prevent the formation of wrinkles.

Obtain fatty acids from cold-pressed vegetable oils. Avoid saturated and animal fats.

*Supermarkets are the problem.* You cannot walk into a supermarket without being bombarded by corn puffs, cheese curls, potato chips, colas, sweets, and readymade foods. If you enter a supermarket on an empty stomach, forget it - any good intentions of buying healthy foods go right out the window. The smells, layout, and design of the supermarket work against your good intentions. When going to the supermarket, follow these guidelines.

1. Go on a medium to satisfied stomach. On an empty stomach, you are more likely to purchase sweets and fatty foods. A full stomach can make you lethargic and easily frustrated.

2. Write down your grocery list on a pad or key it into your cell phone.

3. Get what you need and leave. Walking around the supermarket increases the likelihood of giving in to temptation.

*Foods to invest in*:

Take stock of your fridge and note the foods you like to eat. Then compare them with the list below. The purpose is to get you to change your eating habits and become healthier.

***Meats***

Chicken - good source of protein, which helps to maintain lean muscle. Chicken is easier to digest than red meats.

Turkey - like chicken, a good source of protein. Turkey contains tryptophan, which induces calmness and sleep. It is also easier to digest than red meats.

Fish - salmon and mackerel. Known for their fatty acids, such as omega 3, which is great for the skin, heart, hair, nails, and arteries, fish are much easier to digest than red meats. Limit consumption to once a week.

## *Vegetables*

**These vegetables contain vitamin A and C, folate, calcium, and copper:**

- Broccoli
- Spinach
- Collards
- Bell pepper
- Kale
- Dandelion greens
- Brussels sprouts
- Peas
- Winter squash
- Swiss chard

Cauliflower has vitamin C, B1, B2, B3, B6, and folate. For people with diabetes, cauliflower is better than cabbage. It also slows down certain cancers.

Tomatoes - contain vitamin C and phytochemicals that are good for the skin. Should be eaten raw as well as cooked. When cooked, tomatoes release lycopene, a powerful antioxidant that destroys free radicals.

Wax, green, and snap beans - these contain vitamin C, vitamin B1, B3, B6, and vitamin E.

Carrots - carrots have a high amount of vitamin A and C, folate, calcium, and copper.

Sweet potatoes - these have a high amount of vitamin A and C, folate, calcium, and copper.

Cabbage - cabbage kills bacteria and viruses, and also controls hormone levels. Good for eczema and other skin rashes. Contains vitamin C, B6, and phytochemicals.

Romaine lettuce - two cups contain 50% of the daily recommended amount of vitamin A. Romaine lettuce also contains vitamin C, vitamin B1, B2, B6, and vitamin E as well.

Beet greens - these contain vitamin C, vitamin E, vitamin B6, B1, and folate acid, which protects against birth defects.

### *Fruits*

Apples - these are good for inflammation and have properties that fight cancer. They contain vitamin B6, vitamin C, folate, and vitamin E.

Apricots - good for the skin, heart, and nerve tissue. They contain B vitamins, vitamin C, folate, and copper.

Avocado - rich in B vitamins and great for the skin. Avocadoes contain monounsaturated fats.

Blueberries - blueberries are antioxidant-rich, great for the skin and slows down the aging process by protecting the cells from free radicals. Blueberries also contain B vitamins, vitamin C, and vitamin E.

Cantaloupe - cantaloupe is great for the skin; it is high in folate, and contains zinc, copper, B vitamins, and vitamin E. It has anti-inflammatory and anti-tumor properties.

Cranberries - these berries are good for bladder, kidneys, and the skin. They stops E. coli from attaching to the bladder. They are rich in vitamin C and contain B vitamins, zinc, and vitamin E.

***Grains***

Brown rice is the best of all varieties of rice. A serving contains 7 grams of protein and provides essential vitamins and minerals. One of its components is fiber, which helps with digestion. White rice and other varieties of rice attach to your small intestine and can stay there for a day or more, slowing the digestion process and promoting weight gain.

Whole grain noodles - these typically contain more protein and dietary fibers that aids digestion. They also have less fat than traditional noodles.

Whole grain bread - this contains grains and fibers that facilitate digestion. If your gluten intolerant purchase gluten free breads.

# Exercise

Exercise is great for the skin. Cardio-based workouts are especially good for maintaining healthy, beautiful skin; the sweat generated from working out cleans the pores of the skin. Working out also circulates blood more quickly to various parts of the body and provides essential nutrients.

Exercising your skin itself is also a good idea. Your skin can not lift weights: however, you can sit in a slanted position upside down for 10 to 15 minutes a day. This helps to take the pull of gravity off your skin and send more nutrients to facial cells. Also, try adding MSM to your diet. After drinking the supplement, wait 10 to 15 minutes, then lay slanted. This will send the MSM particles to your facial skin faster and maximize the effectiveness of both MSM and the slanted technique.

# Avoid These Things

Do not smoke! Smoking dries out your skin, and has numerous negative effects on your health that lead to premature aging and even death. If you have the urge to smoke, chew on carrots or lollipops instead.

Alcohol and caffeine should also be avoided they dry out the skin, which makes it susceptible to wrinkling. Red wine is one alcohol that can be consumed because it contains antioxidants, but it should only be used in moderation (once or twice week).

Your facial expressions - believe it or not - also contribute to fine lines and wrinkles. If you squinting, cringing, scowling, and even raising your eyebrows excessively, can cause lines and wrinkles to form, especially if skin is dry or dehydrated.

# NUTRITIONAL SUPPLEMENTS

Did you know that it takes at least 5 servings of vegetables and fruits each day to obtain the recommended amount of nutrients? Who has the time to eat 5 servings of fruits and vegetables daily? Many experts in the past have said you can get all your vitamins and minerals through your daily diet. But for many of us who have busy lifestyles, this is not possible. In addition, much of our soil is depleted of essential minerals, which means they are absent from our foods. Thus, we should replace these minerals through supplementation.

Nutritional supplements come in the form of pills, powders, liquids, sublinguals, and sometimes injections, which should be performed by a health care professional. Besides injections, using sublinguals, which are placed under the tongue, is usually the fastest way to activate supplements in the body, followed by liquids, powders, and then pills. Nutritional supplements include **vitamins, minerals, hormones, herbs, phytochemicals, essential fatty acids, amino acids**, and **prescribed drugs**.

*Important supplements:*

MSM (2000-3000mg) - strengthens skin and hydrates skin cells.

Vitamin A (5,000-20,000 IU) - great for acne and wrinkles.

Vitamin B (complex 50mg) - great for all skin disorders.

Essential fatty acids/primrose/black currant (1000mg 3 times daily).

Carnosine (100-400mg) prevents sugars from bonding with fats and proteins which create  substances that damages the skin and other tissue

Zinc (50mg for men, 100mg for women, plus copper 5) - make sure you eat enough.

Kelp (1000-1500mg) - promotes good skin tone.

Selenium (200mcg) - works with vitamin C as a free radical scavenger.

Vitamin C ester (500-1500mg per day recommended) - repairs skin and strengthens with collagen.

Vitamin C (ascorbic with fish oil) - keeps the body from getting accustomed to the ester C form. Fish oil will allow the vitamin C to stay in your system longer.

Vitamin E (400mg) - heals and repairs skin.

Vitamin D3 (400-800mg) - skin cells use this to regenerate, essential for people who stay mostly indoors.

Calcium magnesium - helps the body absorb zinc and strengths skin.

Flaxseed oil (1000mg daily) - helps to lubricate the skin.

Grape seed extract (as prescribed) - fights free radicals.

Superoxide dismutase (SOD) (as prescribed on label) - take with vitamins C and E for optimal effect.

***Minerals:***

Calcium - great for growing and maintaining health bones; keeps the skin healthy.

Chromium - good for fighting cross-glycosylation and balancing sugar levels. Consult with a physician before using this supplement, because everyone has a different requirement for this mineral.

Copper - an important element that helps with the formation of elastin and collagen, both elastin and collagen are responsible for making the skin supple and youthful. Consult a physician before using. Do not use more than 3 milligrams daily. Take with 50mg of zinc.

Potassium - potassium deficiencies are linked to acne. Stress increases the need for potassium.

Selenium - a powerful antioxidant that works synergistically with vitamin E. It also helps aid the function of the skin's elastin.

Silicon - this comes in a form know as silica, which is great for your skin, hair and nails. Use a silica product that does not contain antacids, which can cause kidney stones. The benefits of this mineral for the skin are too often overlooked. Silicon slows down the aging process and prevents wrinkles. It stimulates collagen and strengthens the skin.

Sulfur - the name does not do it justice; it sounds like a harmful chemical. But sulfur performs some important bodily functions. It protects the body against toxic substances and slows down the aging process. It is also needed for the synthesis of collagen. MSM is a good source of sulfur.

Zinc - prevents acne by regulating oil glands. It is necessary for healing wounds and the synthesis of collagen. It also fights free radicals.

***Herbs:***

Acerola hydrates the skin.

Alfalfa, borage oil, burdock root, chamomile, horsetail, oat straw, red raspberry, and thyme are all good for general nourishment of the hair, skin, and nails.

Aloe vera has soothing, healing, and moisturizing properties. Apply pure aloe vera gel to dry skin as directed on the product label.

Comfrey is good for alleviating dry skin.

Borage seed, cranberry, flaxseed, ginger root, lavender, lemongrass, parsley, and pumpkin seed are also good for toning the skin.

To control melanin production, use alpha lipoic acid, green tea, idebenone, super oxide dismutase, and vitamins E.

**Recap**

Vitamins A, B, C, and E are most important for the skin. Zinc, selenium, calcium, and magnesium are vital minerals for skin health and anti-aging. Hormones that are important for anti-aging are melatonin, DHEA, and HGH (human growth hormones). The herbs that are essential for slowing down the aging process are acerola, calendula, comfrey, green tea, noni, witch hazel, and acai. Phytochemicals come from plant sources and can be found in foods such as brussel sprouts, cauliflower, cabbage, tomatoes, green tea, blueberries, bilberries, and citrus fruits. Essential fatty acids responsible for anti-aging are primrose oil, black current oil, omega 3, 6, and 9, flaxseed oil, and cod liver oil. The essential amino acids are L-Arginine, L-Lysine, L-Tyrosine, and L-Ornithine. The medicines that reduce wrinkles are Botox and Retin A, a form of vitamin A.

# Facial Care

### *Skin care/topical creams*

Many cosmetic companies spend millions of dollars a year on facial products. If you think those expenses go into research of the actual creams, you are sadly mistaken. The majority of that money goes into the package design of the product. If you walk into the cosmetic section of any retail store, you will see hundreds of over-priced bottles of face lotion, potions, and other cosmetics in beautifully designed bottles. The colors range from ultraviolet pink to radiant orange to sky blue. At times I am tempted to buy some of these products, even with my knowledge of their chemical makeup. The truth is, the contents in most of these fancy bottles will not make your skin any more beautiful.

### *Face wash*

As far as soaps go, use a gentle soap that isn't going to strip away the natural oils of the skin. Use mild liquid soaps that do not strip the moisture from the skin. Your face wash should also be free of detergents. Soaps that foam contain detergents. Ingredients to Look for:

Glycerin - used in soap to hold in moisture

Salicylic acid- sheds away dead skin cells

### *Exfoliation*

Some experts say you should exfoliate every day, others say once a week. Some say don't exfoliate at all. The truth is: you should exfoliate two to three times a week. When you exfoliate, make sure your skin has no flare-ups or open wounds. Use a gentle exfoliate that has a liquid base. Recent research suggests that loofahs are too abrasive for facial tissue and can cause inflammation by rupturing the skin's surface. For manual exfoliates a washcloth or a facial sponge rubbed in circular motion are good options. However, sponges retain bacteria that can infect the skin and cause inflammation. Therefore, if used, sponges should be bought in small pieces or cut into small pieces and after every use disposed of. For liquid exfoliates alpha hydroxy acids are great, they tighten the skin, reduce fine lines and wrinkles, and facilitates in the brightening of the skin; try dermaE's *Alpha Hydroxy Acids Beauty Fluid,* for use follow as directed.

### *Toner*

When should you use a toner? There are two main types of toners: astringents and moisturizing toners. Astringents strip away oil from the skin. This helps to reduce the formation of acne. Moisturizing toners moisturize the skin and serve as a base for moisturizer. Toners are also used for toning and complexion enhancement of the skin.

All toners are not made equal. Many contain alcohol, which dries the skin, and other chemicals, which can cause irritation. Toners range in price from $8.00 to $40.00. Witch hazel is a good natural toner that cleanses the skin.

Tone: A salicylic acid formula once or twice a day reduces oil and clear pores. (One to try: Clean & Clear Oil Controlling Astringent.) Apply with a cotton ball, concentrating on T-zone: forehead, nose, and chin.

Witch hazel - natural astringent that tones skin.

Cucumber - has amino and organic acids that soothe and tighten skin.

Chamomile - good for sensitive skin, an anti-inflammatory, and anti-bacterial.

Burdock - eliminates poisons from the skin.

Arnica - repairs skin. An astringent with soothing capabilities.

Reminder: moisturizing tonners moistens the skin and astringent toners tend to dry the skin and treat acne.

## *Moisturizers*

The goal of moisturizers is to help lipids hold in moisture. People who take cholesterol drugs may suffer from dry skin; that is why they need essential fatty acids. Moisturizers should contain both occlusive and humectants ingredients. Humectants ingredients grab moisturizer out of the air and occlusive ingredients lock in moisture. Other ingredients to look for in Moisturizers:

Allantoin - a soothing agent derived from comfrey.

Aloe vera - rich in nutrients and softens the skin.

Aspartic acid - used to enhance skin smoothness.

Calendula - promotes tissue growth, soothes and softens sensitive skin.

Comfrey - heals irritated skin.

Essential fatty acids - repair and lubricate skin.

Ginko biloba - circulates oxygen to skin, also an anti-oxidant that makes skin look younger.

Glycerin - used in soap to hold in moisture.

Ivy - helps with circulation and allows other ingredients to penetrate the skin.

Liposome - helps carry ingredients deep into the skin.

Panthenol - moisturizes and soothes irritation.

Retionic acid - a form of vitamin A that improves circulation and smoothes out skin.

Sage - helps relieve dry, itchy skin.

Yarrow - anti-inflammatory that tightens skin.

Hyaluronic acid - moisturizes the skin; molecules are too big to pass through pores.

DMAE cream - has been shown to increase the skin firmness.

Peptides - boost collagen.

Ester C - face cream from Jason's.

Vitamin A - an effective face cream.

Collagen cream - a good moisturizer, use as prescribed.

Elastin cream - use as prescribed.

*Always treat the main skin types first which you could also treat with one sub-skin type at a time.*

# Suggested Regimens

*Dry skin*

**Face Wash:** Use pure avocado, olive, or almond oil. Rub a small amount on your face then rise off with warm water.

*Alternative*: Wash face in cool to cold-water using use Jason's Ester C Cleanser.

**Toner:** Use lavender water.

**Moisturizer:**

*Day and Night Use*: 4 times a week or more

Mix Vitamin A gel (5 to 8 squeezes) with an Ester C capsule (500mg), stir or shake until it liquefies and then add Vitamin A & E oil (pour 7 to 10 drops) to the contents. Mix contents in a small darkly colored spray bottle.

*Nighttime* Use: 2 to 3 times a week

Collagen cream

Or

Hyaluronic acid

### *Oily skin*

**Face Wash:** Use E-Gem Skin-Care soap (contains vitamin A & E) wash using warm to very warm water.

**Toner:** Use tea tree oil-water: 30ml of distilled mixed with 4to 6 drops of tea tree oil, if skin becomes too dry or tight, switch to Lavender water or witch hazel.

**Moisturizer:** In your hand mix Vitamin A Gel, tea tree oil-water, and Lavender water then apply.

*Alternative*: Mix vitamin C and Zinc with distilled water (spritz on face, 1 to 3 times daily)

Also, use talcum power after applying moisturizer because it evens out excess moisture. Make sure your face is clean before applying.

### *Combination skin*

*Reminder*: The T-zone is usually oily and the cheeks are either normal or dry. In addition, vitamin A facial gel can be used on your entire face because it is grease-free.

**Face Wash:** Use *Carlson's E Gem Skin Care* soap on oily areas wash-off using warm water. For normal or dry areas, wash in cool to cold-water using use Jason's Ester C Cleanser.

**Toner:** Use witch hazel or Lavender water is good for all main skin types. For excessive oiliness, use tea tree-oil solution on those areas only.

**Moisturizer:**

*Oily areas*: In hand mix DermaE Vitamin A Moisturizing gel, tea tree oil water (2 sprays), and lavender water (2 sprays) and apply.

*Dry or normal areas*: Spray on the mixture of Vitamin A gel with Ester C

Use talcum powder on nose or on areas of the face that produces the most oil.

### *Pigmented skin*

**Face Wash:** Use the face wash recommended for your main skin type

**Toner:** Lemon oil mixed with lavender water

*Alternative*: Use over the counter toners that contain soy or niacinamide ingredients.

**Moisturizer:** Use Retinol A with vitamin E.

*Alternative*: Use Retinol A individually, and add a small amount of vitamin E directly to marked areas. In addition, camellia and/or flaxseed oil can be rubbed directly on scars.

Make sure to use sunblock or sunscreen after using, soy, niacinamide, or Retinol A products, because these products make the skin more sensitive to sunlight.

### *Thin/Wrinkled skin*

**Face wash:** Use pure avocado, olive, or almond oil then wash-off with warm water. Or use a mild soap (containing vitamin A & E).

**Toner:** Distilled water mixed with vitamin C (keep cold) or lavender water.

**Moisturizer:** Mix Vitamin A gel (5 to 8 squeezes) with an Ester C capsule (500mg), stir or shake until it liquefies and then add Vitamin A & E oil to the contents. (Mix contents in a small darkly colored spray bottle)

Use Hyaluronic acid or collagen creams two to three times a week at night.

Elastin cream-Put directly on wrinkles at least three to four times a week at night. Use in conjunction with the moisturizers mentioned above.

### *Sensitive skin*

**Face wash**: Use the face wash recommend for your main skin type.

Also, consider washing with pure avocado oil or use a mild, fragrance-free soap that contains no preservatives.

**Toner**: Use lavender water or witch hazel- test on small areas of your skin first to test sensitivity.

**Moisturizer**:

*Dry sensitive skin*: use pure Avocado oil mixed with vitamin E

*Oily sensitive skin*: use vitamin A gel mixed with vitamin C (spritz on and then rub in).

### *Acne*

**Face wash:** Use E Gem soap, wash in warm water.

**Toner:** Use tea tree oil-water: 30ml of distilled mixed with 4to 6

drops of tea tree oil

*Alternative*: Use a products that contains benzoyl peroxide.

**Moisturizer:** Mix Vitamin A Gel, tea tree oil-water (2 sprays), with Lavender water (2 sprays) then apply.

### *Things to keep in mind*

Use witch Lavender or water hazel to tone the skin. Do not use products containing alcohol because they dry the skin.

# Homemade Treatments for Skin

There are many excellent home facial treatments that can help with specific skin problems. Some of the best include:

To rejuvenate the skin and give it a glow, mash 4 to 5 of strawberries together and then apply them to your face. Leave them on for six to eight minutes, and then rinse with lukewarm water.

If you have puffiness or dark circles around the eyes, place cucumber slices or a cold spoon over your eyes for ten minutes or longer if needed.

To exfoliate or take away dead skin, take a handful of rice or oat meal and rub it over your face in a circular motion for 3 to 5 minutes. Use a large bowl because the rice has a tendency to scatter.

To stimulate collagen and exfoliate your skin, mash together 2 to 4 grapes and rub it on your face apply it to your face while you relax, and then rinse it off. Leave on for 10 minutes.

Wrinkle prevention: mash half or a whole of a small avocado and apply it to your face. Leave it on between 20 to 30 minutes, then rise off with lukewarm water. Especially good for those with dry skin.

To decrease excess oils and firm up skin, take one or two eggs and extract the white. Whip it up in an bowl then apple to face for fifteen to twenty minutes, rinse it off with warm water.

Put light oils on around the eye area before bed time such as Derma E Vitamin A with E oil, before going to bed.

# Sunblock/Sunscreen

Protection from the sun's rays is essential to reduce aging of the skin and prevent other damage. Sunblock and sunscreen are terms used interchangeably these days. The precise definition for sunblock is a substance that blocks the sun's rays and contains zinc oxide and titanium dioxide. It is not very absorbable, and preferable because it is less irritating and not as dangerous for the skin compared to sunscreens. Sunscreen is a cream that binds to the skin and absorbs sunlight. Ideally, you should wear sunblock; sunblock is better than sunscreen because it interacts less with your skin and causes less photo damage.

No matter what your age or skin type, you must protect yourself from the sun. Always apply sunblock or sunscreen, preferably with a skin protection factor (SPF) of at least 15 to 25; apply to all exposed areas of the skin between the hours of 8 am and 4 pm, regardless of the weather or the season. Sun exposure is the greatest source of skin damage and biological aging of the skin. Because of their chemical makeup, most if not all sunscreens can damage your skin. Every skin care expert encourages the use of sunscreen, but doesn't tell you the dangers associated with the chemicals contained in these sunscreens. They can cause cancer as well as photo aging. That is why it is important to have a protective barrier on your skin between sunscreens.

Follow these guidelines for optimal use of sunscreen and sunblock:

1. Buy sunblock that contains zinc oxide and/or titanium oxide, which protects against both UVA and UVB rays. Zinc oxide and titanium oxide are less irritating to the skin than their chemical

counterparts. Avoid sunscreens that contain PABA or para-aminobenzoic acid.

2. If you are extremely fair and burn easily, Avobenzone offers the best protection against UVA rays; however, it can irritate and cause damage to the skin. Only use products containing Avobenzone if it doesn't irritate your skin. If irritation occurs, discontinue use.

3. For any sunscreen, with the exception of natural oils such as avocado or coconut oil, remember to create a barrier between your skin and the sunscreen with a moisturizer. If you have dry skin, use an oil-based moisturizer. Make sure you give your skin 3 to 5 minutes to absorb the moisturizer before applying sunscreen. You can also add capsules of vitamin A, C, and E to your moisturizer to further create a barrier between your skin and to counteract potential damage the sunscreen may cause. If you have dark skin, you may be able to use avocado oil as sunscreen.

4. Avoid products that contain PABA or para-aminobenzoic acid, which have a high rate of skin irritation. Your sunblock should contain zinc oxide and titanium dioxide.

5. Wear a hat and tightly woven clothes. Also, make sure you have a pair of wide eye sunglasses.

6. Make sure you apply sunscreen to face, neck, chest, hands, and back; anywhere that is exposed to the sun, especially if you are fair-skinned.

7. If you are in the sun between the hours of 8 am and 4 pm, wear a sun protection factor of 45 or more.

8. After you come home, wash off your sunscreen (assuming it is after 4pm).

If the methods and suggestions in this book are followed, your skin will greatly improve, guaranteed. Existing wrinkles will decrease, and your skin will glow and be much more vibrant.

# Allergens and the Skin

Once I was working with a customer who was taking several supplements to improve her mood and overall skin vitality. The client complained about a rash that wasn't going away. I asked her when the rash appeared, what kind of food she was eating, and if she had recently changed her diet in any way. After ruling out several possibilities, I asked her what supplements she was taking. She read down the list: vitamin C, B, B12, St. John's wort... I stopped her there and told her to stop using the herb for a week. The rash cleared right away. St. John's wort was the culprit, and causes allergic reactions in some people.

It's important to pay attention to your body and be aware of your health. The bottom line is, if you're not healthy, you're not going to look good, period. Once I made a vegetable drink with tomatoes, carrots, and kale. I drank it and after felt terrible. I thought to myself, I just drank this youth serum and now I look worse because of it. A day later, I realized the tomatoes were spoiled.

Allergens are lurking all around us: in our food, our homes, and everywhere outside. When preparing vegetable and fruit juices, make sure you thoroughly wash all fruits and vegetables (often they have wax or in-pesticides on the outside). When possible, try to eat organic fruits and vegetables to prevent the likelihood of wax or pesticide contamination. If an apple is not organically grown, peel the skin to prevent consumption of pesticides.

***Vitamins*** should be stored in a cool, dry place unless the instructions say otherwise. Liquids are usually stored in the fridge. Fish oil in soft gel form can be stored in the freezer to prevent fishy odor of your breath after consumption (you can also get flavored fish oil). Look at the date the products were manufactured. In the past, products would list an expiration date, but now regulations have changed. The latest manufactured supplements list the manufacture date instead of the expiration date.

*Internal & External Starvation*

There are many weight loss programs and diets that require you to restrict caloric intake and deprive you of certain food groups, such as carbohydrates. This can be a major issue. Your body needs a significant amount of carbohydrates to think and maintain a balanced mood. The skin needs fats (lipids), water (moisture), and protein. If you do not eat a significant amount of food, your skin will get dull. Preexisting lines can start to become more pronounced within 10 to 24 hours of not eating. Starving for nourishment, your body will start to use up its reserves of stored fats, which can produce needed oil for your skin.

I am not encouraging you to overeat or binge on junk foods. However, I am encouraging you to eat sufficient amounts of healthy food for optimal skin health. Check the Diet section for further details.

Starving your skin externally means not giving it the nourishment it needs to be healthy, vibrant, and radiant by using topical care products. Topical care products are facial soaps, oils, toners, moisturizers, serums, and sunscreen. Using the correct facial cleanser clears pores and leaves natural oil in the skin. Facial soaps help toners and moisturizers to nourish the skin by removing dead skin and other debris. Astringent-based toners are used to tighten pores, reduce oil, and kill bacteria. Toners with a moisturizer-base and moisturizers are used to moisten skin and supply it with nutrients such as vitamins, minerals, and antioxidants. It is essential to give your skin the supplements it needs to ensure beauty and longevity.

# Antioxidants

Antioxidants are nutrients that fight oxidation. Oxidation occurs when the body goes about performing its normal functions, even mundane ones, such as breathing or digesting food. The oxidation process produces free radicals that destroy the body's healthy cells and wreak havoc on its organs. In addition, oxidation damage can occur from exposure to smoking, environmental pollutants, and fried foods to name a few. However, anti-oxidants combat free radicals and protect the body from oxidation damage. Different antioxidants work differently to combat different forms of oxidation.

Below is a list of antioxidants that help fight aging and protect the skin!

Alpha lipoic acid--Enhances the effectiveness of vitamin E, vitamin C, and COQ 10. It also balances sugar levels in the blood.

Bilberry - lowers blood sugar levels and is stronger than vitamin E and Vitamin C. It increases the strength of collagen and is an anti-inflammatory. It is also great for the eyes.

Burdock root - fights hydrogen peroxide and superoxide radicals, and increases the effectiveness of vitamin E. May help protect cell form destruction.

Carotenoids - found in carrots, carotene is a form of carotenoids, and they have antioxidant effects.

Coenzyme Q 10 - contained in skin cells, good for circulation of nutrients to the skin.

Curcumin (Turmeric) - an herb with anti-inflammatory properties. It stops the formation of free radicals and kills existing ones.

Flavonoids - protects vitamins from becoming damaged by oxidation and attaches itself to metals to stop their harmful effects on the body.

Garlic -protects the body from oxidation and free radical damage. Aged garlic protects against sun damage.

Ginko Biloba - helps to circulate blood, which is necessary for the skin to receive nutrients.

Glutathione - protects cells from free radical damage, such as radiation form chemotherapy, cigarette smoke, and alcohol. Protects the skin and has other anti-aging benefits. Seek medical advice before taking this supplement.

Green tea -protects DNA in the skin. It also has anti bacterial and antiviral properties, it also helps to regulate sugar levels. Good to add in skin creams.

Methionine - destroys the most serious free radicals and protects the skin form the sun's rays. (May cause brain damage if used in excess amounts.)

N-Acetylcysteine (NAC) - slows cellular damage related to aging and cleans body of pollutants. Consult a physician before using; could interfere with insulin production.

Nicotinamide adenine dinucleotide (NADH) - repairs and maintains

DNA in cells.

Oligomeric proanthocyanidins/pycnogenol - protects the brain and central nervous system from oxidative damage, and strengthens and repairs connective tissue in the skin. It also slows down the aging process and decreases inflammation response to allergens by decreasing the amount of the hormone histamine.

Silymarin - derived from milk thistle, protects the liver from oxidative damage.

Sodium oxide dismutase - must be absorbed in the small intestine. Fights free radicals that destroy synovial fluid, and decreases inflammation.

Vitamin A - smooths out the skin and reduces wrinkles. Also protects cells from oxidation

Vitamin E - circulates blood and takes nutrients to skin. It is also an antioxidant that works with selenium to destroy free radicals.

Vitamin C - helps stimulate collagen production, reduces fine lines and wrinkles. Protects against various forms of free radicals.

Zinc - repairs skin, regulates oil glands, and is a powerful antioxidant.

Selenium - works hand-in-hand with vitamin E to protect skin tissue and cell membranes. Also protects the body from hydrogen peroxide.

# Stretch Marks

Stretch marks happen when your body grows or enlarges, which causes tissue to expand, stretching the skin. Stretch marks are caused by pregnancy, sudden weight gain, and weight lifting. They can appear on the breast, buttocks, stomach, shoulders, and biceps.

Vitamin E is great for stretch marks: apply it to the affected area consistently for thirty days, and you should see a diminished amount of stretch marks. Also, cocoa butter is a good way to get rid of stretch marks.

# Age Spots

Age spots are also called liver spots; they are cauterized by flat brown spots that can vary in size. Age spots can surface anywhere on the body, but mostly appear on the face, neck, and hands. Age spots are usually harmless, but some spots may be cancerous, or highlight a problem, that is why it is important for a dermatologist to examine all spots on the skin. Age spots occur from the combination of waste, free radicals, and sun exposure. They mirror what is going on in the cell of your body.

To minimize the formation of age spots one should eat a healthy diet, exercise, and protect themselves against the sun. Also, poor liver function, and ingestion of fried foods over a period of time, can also lead to age spots. Sun exposure is the main component of age spots, people who have large amount of age spots, usually live in sunny climates. However, diet and nutrition are also important factors.

**Nutritional Supplement/Vitamin and Minerals**

Vitamin A 5000 IU

Vitamin C 2000 mg

Vitamin E 400 mg

Zinc 15-30 mg

Selenium 100 mcg

Super Oxide Dismutase (SOD) Used as prescribed on the label

The above vitamins and supplements help to rejuvenate skin cells and combat oxidative processes that lead to age spots.

*Preventative:*

Wear sun block.

Use cinnamon/cinnamon pills when eating sugary foods to offset the negative effects of sugar.

*Applications*:

Vitamin E oil rub a small amount on age spots or mix vitamin E with Eucalyptus oil and apply to age spot.

Rub a small amount of diluted lemon juice on age spots (stop if irritation occurs).

Use soy skin tonners and facial lotions that contain soy ingredients.

*Reminder:* follow cleansing program *Blood, Kidney, & Liver* in chapter 7. A through cleanse is essential in preventing and getting rid of age spots.

# Aromatherapy for the Skin

Aromatherapy was used by the ancient Greeks, Indians, and Egyptians, which would explain the glowing and flawless skin of those ancient people. These oils are either massaged onto the skin, put in bath water, ingested orally, or inhaled. Instead, we are going to focus on these oils as they relate to the improvement of your skin. They can be used for acne, dry skin, oily skin, mature skin, psoriasis, burns, and sunburns. Use these natural blends as a supplemental program to your beauty regimen.

**Acne** *Astringent*

| | |
|---|---|
| Distilled Water | 30 ml |
| Tea tree oil | 3 drops |
| Lavender oil | 1 drop |

Start with mild dosages and increase as needed

**Dry Skin** *Toner*

| | |
|---|---|
| Distilled Water | 30 ml |
| Lavender oil | 2 drops |
| Frankincense oil | 1 drop |

**Combination Skin** *Moisturizer*

| | |
|---|---|
| Jojoba oil | 30 ml |
| Rose oil | 2 drops |
| Neroli oil | 2 drops |
| Palmarosa oil | 2 drops |

**Thin/wrinkled skin** *Moisturizer*

| | |
|---|---|
| Jojoba oil | 30 ml |
| Frankincense oil | 2 drop |
| Helichrysum oil | 2 drop |
| Rose oil | 3 drops |

In several weeks you will see great improvement in your skin.

(Note: store these mixtures in the fridge.)

# Conclusion

There is a wide range of cosmetic procedures that can be done. These procedures include facial peels, cosmetic skin surgery, laser resurfacing, Botox injection, collagen injection, and hyaluronic acid injection are some of the things that can be done by a licensed dermatologist. However, be sure to exhaust all natural methods recommended before investing in cosmetic procedures. Natural methods are safer and more cost effective.

Caucasian women are more suited for cosmetic procedures, especially those with fairer complexions. Healing after procedures causes little to no scarring in these women, because of the reduced amounts of melanin in their skin. However, African American women after such procedures would scar more easily because of the melanin content in their skin.

Following the directions in this book could stop or even prevent the need for cosmetic surgeries. I guarantee you that your skin will improve beyond your expectations. These are all-natural and proven scientific methods for young and healthy skin. If you have any questions pertaining to this book, please send me an email at wrinkleprevention@gmail.com.

# Anti-Wrinkle Glossary

Acidophilus - good bacteria that fights infection, inflammation, and other bad bacteria such as candidiasis

Alpha hydroxy acid - diminishes fine lines and wrinkles through exfoliation and helps skin look smother

Alpha lupoic acid - powerful anti-aging agent, balances sugar levels and decreases cross-glycosation

Aluminum - an ingredient in deodorant that can cause significant harm to the body; it is also associated with Alzheimer's disease

Amino acids - necessary for repairing the skin

Aminobutyric acid - this is an amino acid that keeps in water, it may have anti-inflammatory properties

Ammonium chloride - an additive to nonalcoholic toners, used to create tingling, stinging sensation

Ammonium cocoyl isethionate - derived from coconut oil, softens skin

Ammonium lactate - derived from lactic acid; makes top layer of the skin thicker and reduces the thickness of the corneum

Ammonium lauryl sulfate - a skin-irritating emulsifier

Ammonium polyacryldimethyltauraminde - a skin thickener with a high PH necessary for water-soluble sunscreen

Amniotic fluid - studies suggest it may have wound-healing and cellular regeneration abilities

Amyl cinnamal - naturally occurring fragrance in some plants, but in cosmetics it comes from a synthetic source

and wrinkles

Anemone extract - has anti-inflammation properties and can heal wounds; certain forms can cause irritation

Angelic - used to cleanse the blood

Anise extract - a fragrance, can produce a severe skin reaction if applied topically

Antioxidants - scavengers that fight free radicals that damage the skin and speed up the aging process

Apple/apple extract - has malic acid and tartic acid that may help with exfoliation

Apricot kernel oil - high in vitamin E, good moisturizer of skin, has the same properties as almond oil but is less expensive; usually used as a carrier of other ingredients and is quickly absorbed by the skin.

Arachidyl propionate - may be better for dry skin; helps deliver products to skin and leaves a shiny sheen

Areca nut extract - used as an astringent, anti-bacterial, and aromatic agent; strengthens capillaries and may bc ablc to regenerate tissue; usually used in oily skin care products

Argan oil - derived from argan tree; conditions, protects, and moisturizes the skin; composed of tocopherol, phenolic acid, carotenes, and essential fatty acids

Arnica extract - used by patients who undergo plastic surgery to heal faster and to treat acne. It also treats reddened and worn-out skin. Used as an astringent, anti-inflammatory, anticoagulant, circulation-stimulation, and healing. Excessive use may cause irritation and inflammation. Some people are allergic to this plant.

Ascorbyl palmitate - a preservative used for antioxidants in

cosmetics, creams, and lotions; has no know toxicity

Astrocaryum butter - helps the skin retain moisture

Avenobenzone - used in sunscreens; it offers a broad range of protection

Avocado oil - a gentle cleanser, has the ability to penetrate the skin, and provides sun protection; Highest-rated among natural sunscreens by encyclopedia of chemical technology for sunscreen effectiveness

Avocado, peanut, coconut, and olive oil work well - avoid sunscreen chemicals like avenobenzone and others

Babassu oil - good for dry skin; recommended for use in sunscreens

Bacaba pulp oil - contains oleic acid and omega 6 (linoleic acid), used for emollient and moisturizing

Balm mint extract - good for acne and after sun exposure treatments; good for blemishes and sensitive skin, as well as for use as a fragrance

Balm mint oil (lemon balm; Melissa oil) - treats dermatitis and eczema, may cause irritation

Balm of gilead - treats eczema and dry skin

Balsam Peru - treats scabies, eczema, and dermatitis

Baobab (adansonia digitata) - highly emollient and soothing, said to have skin firming ability and the ability to improve the elasticity of the skin

Barberry extract - great for contagious irruptions, is an anti-inflammatory and an antiseptic

Barley oil - a carrier oil, soothes the skin

Basil oil - may be used for acne; stimulates and purifies; works together with methyl chavicol, eucalyptol, linalool, and estragol

Bayberry - can be used for acne and damaged skin

Bean oil - good for acne and reduces itching

Bearberry - anti-inflammatory properties; has the ability to lighten the skin

Beech tree extract - increases protein synthesis and enzymatic activity of keratinocytes; has antiseptic and stimulation qualities, which make it good for treating skin diseases

Beeswax - like petroleum, it forms a network rather than a film; may have antioxidant and anti-inflammatory abilities; can cause allergic reactions in cosmetics

Benzoin - a fragrance oil that has bactericidal, anti-irritation and anti-itching properties; maintains fats and reduces skin redness

Benzophenone 2 - ingredient used in sunscreens

Benzophenone 3 (oxybenzone) - absorbs UVAs and UVB rays

Benzophenone 4 (sulisobenzone) - blocks UVA rays, usage levels 5 to 10 percent, anti-photo oxidant

Benzophenone 8 (dioxybenzone) - UVA absorption

Benzoyl peroxide - used to treat acne, wipes away free fatty acids and skin infection, has been known to cause irritation

Benzyl laurate - non-toxic, non-irritating, non-viscous, non-oily emollient ester that leaves skin feeling smooth; decreases the oiliness of mineral oil

Benzyl salicylate - naturally occurring fragrance found in jasmine oil,

Neroli, and ylang-ylang; can also be synthetic

Bergamot oil - treats oily skin and acne, high concentrates of oil can cause irritation

Beta hydroxy acid (BHA) - good for acne and exfoliation of dead skin (stratum corneum thickness); salicylic acid is an example of this

Beta-glucan - stimulates the formation of collagen; used for fine lines and wrinkles

Beta-lipo hydroxy acid -a slightly weaker form of salicylic acid used to prevent acne from reccurring, and improves skin tolerance of Tretinoin, when used with retinoid

BHA (butylated hydroxyanisole) - has antioxidant capabilities and is a preservative

Bilberry fruit extract - an antioxidant with anti-inflammatory properties; protects collagen from degradation. (Bilberry is not only for the eyes.) Contains a flavonoid called anthocyanin, which is also found in grapes, beets, and eggplant. It also protects capillaries and keeps them strong.

Bioflavoniod - flavonoids that are bioactive, they help with the absorption of vitamin C

Bioflavonoid - has antioxidant capabilities, absorbs oxygen radicals that cause skin oxidation; also antimicrobial, which helps with anti-inflammatory actions

Biotin - good for acne, may have healing properties. Its internal effects on skin are known, but effectiveness of topical application is unclear.

Birch bark extract - anti-irritant, anti-septic properties; treats acne and eczema, used in aftershaves

Birch leaf extract - may have antiseptic and astringent properties;

aromatic

Bisabolol - has anti-inflammatory and soothing properties; comes from chamomile and/or yarrow

Bismuth oxychloride, mica, and silica - found in cosmetics and skin creams; reduce wrinkles

Bitter almond - may cause irritation and skin reactions

Black currant extract - astringent, has smoothing properties, and may have anti-inflammatory properties

Black currant seed oil - good for dry skin, has fatty, linoleic, and linolenic acid, which when added to the skin, replenishes the skin's oil

Black willow bark extract - has high salicylic acid content, which is why it is used for exfoliation

Blackberry extract -used to treat acne, high in tannin, a good astringent

Blessed thistle - effective for skin problems such as papules and pustules, heals sores and reduces itching

Boldine - has antioxidant properties and blocks against UVB rays

Borage extract - anti-inflammatory, good for sensitive skin and allergic reactions

Boric acid - not good for cosmetic products; may cause rashes and irritations

Boron nitride - used for color, has smooth and slippery qualities

Boxwood - can cause itching and irritation

Burdock root extract - anti-fungal, anti-inflammatory, and anti-bacterial; relieves bruises and is good for acne

Buriti pulp oil - may improve elasticity of skin, emollient, antioxidant, has carotene and essential fatty acids; hyderates the skin; hydrolipid barrier; also good for sunburned skin

Butches broom - anti-itching, slimming and anti-cellulite properties, and is a diuretic

Butyl oleate - an ester of butyl alcohol and oleic acid that moisturizes skin, emollient

Butyl stearate - emulsifier known to cause an allergic reaction

Butyldiadipate - an emollient and pH-adjusting agent with penetration ability

Butylenes glycol - a solvent that has goo antimicrobial action and enhances preservative activity and masks order

Caffeine - breaks down fats and drains the skin; because of this it is used for eye creams, cellulite lotion

Cajeput oil - used for psoriasis and eczema, counterirritant properties, similar to camphor and eucalyptus

Calamine - a mineral solution that treats sunburn and contains zinc oxide

Calamint - reduces bruising

Calcium hydroxide - can burn the skin and eyes

Calcium pantetheine sulfonate - lightens the skin, boosts UV protection from sunscreens, and has anti-inflammatory properties

Calcium thioglycolate - can cause skin irritation

Calophyllum inophyllum seed oil - an antioxidant that can absorb UV rays and has antimicrobial and skin conditioning properties; may be able to regenerate skin cells

Camelina sativa seed oil - said to have the ability to improve elasticity and suppleness of the skin

Camellia oil - non grease, anti-oxidation

Camphor - effective treatment for acne; it is absorbed through the skin, mixes with glucuronic acid and passes through urine; may cause irritation and numb peripheral sensory nerves

Camphor benzalkonium methosulfate - a UV filter and absorber; has antimicrobial properties

Canola oil -emollient and lubricant, natural replacement for mineral oil

Caprylic/capric triglyceride (tricaprylin) - promotes penetration and is non-greasy

Caprylol collagen amino acids - anti-acne treatments

Capryloyl collagenic acid - treats mild acne; acne may reappear

Caraway oil - alleviates bruises, may have the ability to regenerate tissue; beneficial for acne and oily skin; belongs to the group of aromatic, umbelliferous plants, such as anise, cumin, dill, and fennel, characterized by carminative properties; found in dill and cumin oils; may cause allergic reactions and skin irritation

Carboxyethy-y-aminobutric acid - may produce cellular growth; has anti-aging properties

Carcinogen - can cause cancer (do not eat burnt food, it speeds up the aging process by way of carcinogens, which enter the body and create free radicals, which damage tissue and causes the skin to wrinkle)

Carnitine - used in hand and body lotions

Carnitine hydroxcitarate - - helps break down fat stored in the cells more effectively than caffeine, making it beneficial for use in slimming and body-contouring products

Carnosine - antioxidant that works to prevent cellular damage due to free radical activity; boosts immunological function and has anti-aging qualities; may stop cross glycosylation; decreases the overall aging process

Carotene - converted by the body into vitamin A, and depending on what your body needs, has photo-protection properties; skin care products: good for dry and scaling skin

Carotenoids - phytochemicals that function as antioxidants

Chinese medicine - traditional Chinese methods of curing ailments

Chondroitin sulfate - great for premature wrinkles

Cinnamon - helps to regulate blood sugar levels, helpful cross-glucosination

Coconut oil - has sun protectant properties

Coenzyme A - detoxifies substances from body

Coenzyme Q10 - necessary for holding moisture in skin

Dermis - the middle layer of the skin

Digestive enzymes - necessary for breaking down and digesting foods; if foods aren't fully digested, they can become rancid in the body, promoting bacteria growth. They can also cause skin breakouts and lead to more serous diseases.

Dioxane -dangerous substance; a petrochemical known to cause cancer

Elastin cream - reduces fine lines and wrinkles

Endorphin - natural substance in the body that is used to decrease the sensation of pain

Epidermis - the first layer of the skin

Essential fatty acids - lubricates and repairs the skin, and reduces wrinkles; good for heart, joints, and overall health

Fbutyl methoxydibenzoylmethane (BMDM, avobenzone) - broad range protection against UVA rays, an ingredient in sunscreen

Flavonoid - crystalline compounds found in plants that work as antioxidants

Free radicals - harmful substances that destroy skin cells and other body organs

Ginko biloba - antioxidant; great for circulation of vitamins and nutrients through the skin; improves memory and brain functionGrapeseed extract - antioxidant that penetrates the brain barrier, good for fighting antioxidants that destroy skin cells

Glucose - a simple sugar used by the body for energy; excessive amounts can lead to diabetes and cross-glucosination

Gluten - protein contained within grains; may cause a reaction in those who have eczema or dermatitis

Homeopathy - uses herbs, minerals, and animal substances to induce symptoms similar to the illnesses in order to cure the illness ("like cures like")

Humectants - attract water from the atmosphereCactus extract - good for sunburn, insect bites, skin irritations, swelling, and inflammation

Hylauronic acid - the best natural skin moisturizer; holds in the most water. Over-the-counter creams with this ingredient cannot get it to a deep layer of the skin because the molecules are too big.

Hypodermis - the third layer of the skin

Inflammation - the swelling and bruising of tissue in which excess amounts of white blood cells are present

Iodine - great for the skin

Isoflavones - prevent the uptake of estrogen

Lavender oil- Has astringent qualities. Freshens the skin, regulates oil production, and smoothes out discolorations.

Lavender water- All skin types can use lavender water. Formula: 30ml of distilled water and four to five drops of lavender oil in a small spray bottle.

Lipids - fats within the skin

Liposomes - bubbles that take ingredients into the skin

Mal-absorption - inability to absorb nutrients from the intestinal tract

Melanin - responsible for the complexion of the skin; protects it from the sun's rays

Milk thistle - cleanses the blood

MSM - powerful anti-wrinkle agent that pushes water molecules to skin cells, which decreases fine lines

Natural moisturizing factor - oil from the skin

Olive oil - has sun protectant properties

Oxidation - reaction with oxygen and other substances in the body which causes a chemical reaction that produces harmful waste

Peanut oil - has sun protection properties

Petrolatum - a mixture of hydrocarbons that is semi-solid; on the skin, it blocks pores form breathing, use should be avoided

Phthalates - cause hormonal problems in women

Preservatives - benzalkonium chloride, benzethonium chloride, benzoic acid; may cause skin irritation

Primrose oil - great for wrinkles; balances estrogen in women

Probiotics - facilitates growth of good bacteria

Propylene glycol - irritates acne and skin Vitamin A - smoothes and repairs the skin; diminishes fine lines and reduces the appearance of wrinkles

Proteins - a nitrogen-based organic compound the body uses to grow bones and heal and repair the skin's tissue

Red blood cells - circulates oxygen and carbon dioxide in the body

Red pop extract - an astringent that masks order

Red vine extract - anti-inflammatory and anti-itching; used to fix broken or fragile capillaries

Rice starch - used in baby powders, smoothes the skin, and has a protective barrier

RNA - takes genetic information from DNA cells to ribosomes, where they are used to replicate more cells with the use of protein

Roman chamomile oil - different from German chamomile; has healing and tonic properties, may be more effective than German chamomile

Rose hip - astringent, rich in vitamin C; roses hip oil hydrates the skin, cleans wounds, and increase healing

Rose petal extract - mild astringent, also used as a tonic

Sialic acid - found in fruits; part of the alpha hydroxy grapesmix family, used to exfoliate skin

Silica - it is in every part of the body and is responsible for the formation of bones, teeth, and skin; reduces wrinkles and fine lines

Sodium oxide dismutase - powerful antioxidant that destroys free radicals

T cells - lymphocyte that is an important part of the immune system

Tea tree oil- Has anticeptic properties. It reduces inflammation and is used to treat acne and oily skin.

Tea tree oil water- Used for oily skin and acne. Formula 30 ml of distilled water mixed with 3 to for drops of tea tree oil.

Topical - the outermost part of the skin

Trace element - an element that is needed by the body, but in minute amounts

T-zone - the forehead and nose, which are most likely to be oily

Vitamin B -- necessary for all skin conditions, helps with repairing the skin; also helps with the tone and complexion of your skin

Vitamin C - repairs the skin, reduces fine lines and wrinkles; there are two forms of vitamin C: ascorbic acid and ester formulation. Ascorbic may pass out of the body quicker and those with sensitive skin may be irritated by topical use. Ester C formulation is buffered with essential oils, which allows it to stay in your body for a longer period of time, up to 10 times that of ascorbic vitamin C. It is also less like to cause skin irritation if used topically.

Vitamin D - repairs the skin and increases glow

Vitamin E - helps with circulating nutrients to the skin, also aids in repairing the skin

Vitamins - organic substances that the body needs; most vitamins must come from diet and nutritional supplementation

White blood cells - fight bacteria, infection, and disease within the body; help repair broken skin

Wild alum - good for oily skin, an astringent and deodorant

Witch hazel - cleans and tones the skin

Zinc - repairs the skin and balances hormones

Made in the USA
Monee, IL
04 November 2026

67386998R00056